"Kombucha 'tea' as it's called is causing quite a stir. The list of ailments it is purported to cure, according to its fans, is staggering: asthma, eczema, low energy, bad digestion. It clears up your skin, gets rid of wrinkles, and even turns hair (or at least some of it) from gray back to its original color. There are even claims that it rebuilds AIDS-ravaged immune systems and mitigates symptoms of multiple sclerosis."

—Los Angeles Times

"The good will and community that have sprung up around Kombucha may be more potent than the tea's medicinal properties."

—The New York Times

"The demand for it is mushrooming."

—Dan Rather
CBS Evening News

Kombucha
PHENOMENON

The Health Drink Sweeping America

The Tea Mushroom Handbook

Betsy Pryor & Sanford Holst

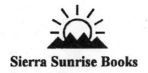

Sierra Sunrise Books

Sierra Sunrise Publishing, Inc.
14622 Ventura Boulevard, Suite 800
Sherman Oaks, CA 91403

Printed in the United States of America
First Printing: July, 1995
Second Printing: September, 1995

Publisher's Cataloging-in-Publication Data

Pryor, Betsy
   Kombucha phenomenon : the health drink sweeping America : the tea mushroom handbook / by Betsy Pryor & Sanford Holst.
   p. cm.
   Includes bibliographical references and index.
   ISBN: 1-887263-10-1

   1. Tea fungus—Therapeutic use. 2. Medicinal plants. I.
Holst, Sanford. II. Title

RM666.T25P79 1995   615'.321
                                   QBI95-20104

Library of Congress Catalog Card Number: 95-68803

Book design by Carolyn Porter and Todd Meisler, One-On-One Book Production and Marketing, West Hills, CA.

Contents

Note

The authors make no claims regarding benefits of the Kombucha mushroom or tea. Always seek the advice of your health care provider.

A few individuals felt their position in life might be jeopardized by revealing they have an illness and chose to use a pen-name; the other names are actual, and all reports of experiences are real.

INTRODUCTION

We made a great discovery in 1993—at least, Betsy Pryor did. Kombucha tea.

I got a surprising phone call from her.

"Listen, I just discovered a great new tea. Makes you feel fantastic!"

"Already drink tea, Betsy. Lipton's"

"Seriously. This is Kombucha tea."

"Come again?"

"A mushroom you put in tea. The tea ferments a little until it tastes like cider."

"You drink this?"

"Every day. And I feel wonderful! You want to try some?"

"Uh . . . sure, Betsy. Eventually."

Come on. I'm a guy who exercises every morning. Why would I need a mushroom?

A few months later, another friend called. She was feeling terrific and doing lots of new things. She started telling me about a mushroom.

"You on this Kombucha thing?" I asked her.

"Yes! Got it from Betsy. Did you get one?"

"Uh, not yet."

Could be just a fad. Probably blow over in a few months.

Then *Los Angeles Magazine* did a fascinating article on people all across the country trying a new Kombucha tea and claiming remarkable results. It featured a woman who had distributed over 3,000 mushrooms. Betsy Pryor.

I picked up the telephone. Had to see a lady about a mushroom.

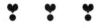

Kombucha tea turns out to be an invigorating health beverage moving past all social barriers in the country. It's used by celebrities and home-makers, active people and couch potatoes, bankers and clerks, and older Americans.

Some people that newspapers and magazines identify as using Kombucha include Daryl Hannah, Ronald Reagan, Rita Coolidge, Madonna, Sharon Farrell, Morgan Fairchild, Linda Evans, Graham Russel and Lily Tomlin.

It's spreading like wildfire. The last time people got this excited was over a new exercise called "aerobics."

Why the excitement?

To tell the truth, the dramatic results people get from drinking Kombucha tea are hard to believe. That's why you won't hear it from us. Instead, we're including a wide sampling of people's personal experiences exactly as they wrote them. Decide for yourself.

People say the tea has helped them with migraine, digestion, skin problems, chemotherapy symptoms, AIDS symptoms, illnesses, insomnia, regularity, T-cell count, multiple sclerosis remission and other effects. One of the great things about the Kombucha mushroom is that it multiplies as it grows. People often give the new mushrooms to friends so they can make their own tea.

How do you make it? It's fairly easy once you know how. Betsy Pryor's method for preparing Kombucha tea is widely acclaimed as the best and safest way. Why mention "safe"? Because it's possible to do it wrong, just like with any other food. All across the country and around the world, people are doing it right. You can too.

Very simply (we go into lots of detail later) a Kombucha mushroom is put into a bowl of tea and sugar. As it grows, the tea ferments. After a week or so, the mushroom is moved to a fresh bowl. Then you drink the mildly-fermented tea.

What's in the tea? Healthy enzymes, organic acids, vitamins and other good things. It's all explained, along with references to long, scientific names that get technical people excited. The "mushroom" that makes the tea is a combination of healthy bacteria and yeast—and though we don't recommend that people eat it, some do. Normally, you just drink the tea.

The story of where Kombucha came from is long and rich with images from many countries, as you will see. The important thing is: what does it do now that it's here?

The excited reactions of people across America reveal the answer. They share their vivid experiences with family members, neighbors, old friends and people they just met. It's the talk of the country.

We'll go into all that.

Betsy Pryor remembers the journey that made her care about people's health and Kombucha. It began, oddly enough, on a trip to Liberia, West Africa in January of 1981.

It was early evening. Humid. Hot as hell. Rainy season was coming. I sat in the bar of Julia's Hotel in what passed for downtown Monrovia, nursing a Fanta and waiting for a friend to return from flying the body of a local official back to his village deep in the bush. I stared at the spatter of bullet holes crazy-quilted across the wall behind the bar while I listened to the conversation of two American geologists a couple of stools down. They were drinking local beer and talking about some mysterious thing called the "Black Rose." I leaned closer. Seems it was a new venereal disease. Left purplish sores that looked like rose petals on the limbs of its victims. "A Lebanese bar girl down the street died from it today," one of the guys whispered. I put down my Fanta with a clunk and moved one stool closer.

"Died?" I gasped, thinking of the panic that the herpes epidemic was causing among my very hip friends in the TV business in L.A. "From a venereal disease? She died?"

They took another swig of their beer, then looked at me and nodded in unison. "Yeah. Everybody who gets it dies," one said. "First they get the sores. Then pneumonia. Then…" He made a slicing gesture across his throat. They shook their heads and ordered another round of Club.

I stared blankly up at the ceiling fan slowly slap-slapping against the torpid air, then looked out the open door to the dusty street, where white European and American men, the engineers, geologists and mining experts who populated this far-away place, strolled in the warm African evening with their "special girls." It's over, I thought. It's all over. These guys would go back to the States. Infect their wives. Their girlfriends. I closed my eyes.

I never forgot that night. It was marked on my soul with an indelible blot. By 1983, the "Black Rose" had been given a name. AIDS. Late at night I would lie awake wondering what had happened to the American and European men and their "special girls." How many of the "girls" were dead? How many of the men had brought the disease back home? And what about the blood bankers who'd come to town that muggy African January so long ago, trolling for cheap blood. How many units did they buy? How many were tainted with the yet-to-be-detected virus? Where did those units end up? Who, I wondered, had they infected?

Already a technical writer, I began studying retro-viruses, talking to scientists, physicists and physicians. Off the record, they told me that what we had seen so far was a walk in the park compared to what was to come. My instincts were right, they confided. The new retroviruses would mutate. Become airborne. By the year 2010, with no cure in sight, we could be looking at the end of the human race.

I spent the next three years writing a science thriller about an airborne killer virus—and based its cure on electromagnetic wave therapy invented by a real guy named Royal Rife back in the 1930's. His therapy had worked against cancer. The University of Southern California Medical School had said as much. But Rife was sued three times, his instruments confiscated. And even though he won the lawsuits, he died a broken man, his discovery swallowed up in the morass of the American legal system.

In August of 1993, my novel was finished.

One night at meditation class, pondering yet another rejection letter, I realized Rife might never get his due, nor the people of the planet any help. I silently prayed, "God, if my book isn't gonna go, *please* give me *something, anything* to help people stay well."

A few minutes later, as I was leaving my meditation class, Sister Joan Derry, one of the meditation teachers, bustled out of the kitchen carrying a pancake type thing enclosed in a clear, plastic bag. "Wait," she called, her cherubic face split in a wide grin, "I've got something for you!"

The thing in the bag looked awful. I backed away. "What," I whispered, "*is* it?"

"It's a Kombucha tea mushroom! People drink the tea and they *feel* better." She handed me a faded sheet of paper. "Look at all the stuff it's good for!"

I scanned the sheet. Fixes everything from arthritis to acne to acid stomach to a hundred other things, it said. I handed it back to her. "Snake oil," I declared, having spent the last three years in medical libraries. "*Nothing* can do all that." I paused. "Except God."

"Take the Kombucha anyway. Sister Denise and I decided that if anybody was going to get it out to people, it was going to be you."

"Yeah, right," I thought as I walked out into the night.

After three weeks of drinking Kombucha tea, the acne I'd had since age thirteen was gone. I'd also lost the first of the fifteen pounds I'd put on since high school. I had to admit I looked and felt pretty good.

And since the Kombucha makes a "baby mushroom" every week, in a few months I'd given one to each neighbor on our little canyon cul-de-sac. Everybody else was feeling pretty good, too. Gates and fences were being mended and painted for the first time in a dozen years. My neighbor Joe, who had just turned seventy-one, was spending a lot of time three stories in the air repairing his roof. A second neighbor was spending Sundays hanging off the side of the cliff edging her property, chopping at the brush with a machete. She was sixty-five and starting to look a lot like Doris Day. Another neighbor was showing off the black hairs growing back into his graying ponytail. I thought I was watching the sequel to *Cocoon*. I had to admit. The stuff was working. All right, so I hadn't found a cure for AIDS. But I *did* find something that was helping people keep healthy. And had to do something about it.

In January of 1994, I took Joan and Denise's advice. It *was* time to get Kombucha to people. Three days after the Northridge, California earthquake, I started Laurel Farms—and began sending Kombucha mushrooms all across the country.

Later came the TV, radio, newspaper and magazine excitement. We were on our way.

WHAT'S THE EXCITEMENT ABOUT?

People who use—and swear by—Kombucha tea come from all walks of life. Some of their experiences are presented here, like a series of colorful and moving snapshots.

Their health before trying this experience varied all over the map. Some were in reasonably good shape and wanted to get better. Others had very difficult problems—including multiple sclerosis or cancer—and were looking for anything to give them a chance. We can't give medical opinions. We're not doctors, and it wouldn't be fair to try.

The people quoted here are talking about their own experiences. They come from South Bend, Indiana and Boca Raton, Florida. From New York City and Los Angeles. From Seattle and Berryville, Arkansas.

They come from cities and towns all across America. Maybe yours.

Ralph
Hair Stylist
New York, NY

I couldn't believe how I felt. Like as if my whole body was glowing like a light bulb. I live and work in New York City and it ain't easy!

No problem [now] — I run up subway steps two at a time. I greet and smile at total strangers on the street. Everybody wants to know what drug I'm on!! Ha, little do they know.

Rita Coolidge
Singer

I have to drink the tea every day because it helps my throat when I'm singing a lot. I also find it helps with jet lag. I don't feel tired and have lots of staying power energy.

Mary Ann
Retired
Tucson, Arizona

I can't believe how great the tea is. I have had a stomach malady for 20 years. [After] 3 days of Kombucha (thanks to my neighbor) I am feeling better already. And what an appetite . . . yeah!

Olya
Part-time Artist
Vienna, Virginia

I was born and raised in the former USSR, and I remember visiting my aunt and being treated to a very special sweet-and-sour tangy drink. I just loved it! My aunt kept a glass jar-bottle on her windowsill with a gauze covering the top, so "it" could breathe but no dust or dirt would get in. We affectionately called it "gribok" — little mushroom.

Unfortunately, my mom thought it would be too much work for her to keep one "gribok" at our house; so I had to wait for those infrequent visits to my aunt's.

I've been in this country for 20 years now, and I always thought that "gribok" was one of those things forever lost to me since I left Russia. So when I saw [Kombucha] it was like ... coming home!

Jim
Financial Services
San Francisco, CA

A skin condition on my face was diagnosed as hereditary. I couldn't put enough skin cream on to keep the skin from flaking. Drinking Kombucha and putting it on my face and hands daily has cleaned it up completely.

And, my digestion has improved.

Cancer Interview

Janeau St. Clair Atlas sits on her hospital bed in the City of Hope. In the rooms around her is the quiet struggle of people dealing with chemotherapy and bone marrow transplants in their fight against cancer.

But not in Janeau's room. Her breast cancer is gone. With pink cheeks and bright eyes, she tells her story.

Growing up in Kentucky, no one in my family had cancer. I couldn't believe it when my doctor diagnosed breast cancer in October (1993). And he said it was the worst, most aggressive kind . . . I would probably live only 3 to 6 months.

I thought, "Just take me out and shoot me." I couldn't deal with it.

That lasted a few hours. Then I said, "OK, what am I going to do about it?"

I allowed the lump to be removed, but after the horror stories I'd heard, refused the chemotherapy.

Five months later the lump was back, the size of a grapefruit. I agreed to chemotherapy.

I had started drinking the Kombucha tea.

That, and a very positive attitude, made a small miracle. Each chemotherapy treatment is supposed to take three days for recovery. Each morning, I had no toxic signs and was back to normal. The doctors were amazed.

And the treatment worked. The cancer lump shrank. The 8 affected lymph nodes cleared up. By the time the second lump was removed, I was cancer-free!

We were incredulous. Including the doctors.

To make sure it never came back, I agreed to bone marrow treatment at the City of Hope. The high dose chemotherapy began on Thanksgiving (1994) and lasted five days. Your skin turns yellow, you become toxic, the whites of your eyes turn orange, and skin peels off your hands. Recovery takes about six weeks.

But not me! My skin is pink and feels like a baby, my eyes are clear and white, a tiny bit of skin peeled and my blood cells are normal. Three weeks! I'm going home Monday. The nurses call me the "miracle child."

Sure, I lost my hair, just like with the other chemotherapy. Big deal. It grows back thicker and better.

I want to help other women deal with cancer. To tell them it takes positive thoughts and Kombucha.

There's so many women dying of breast cancer because they're scared of what the treatment is. That's what happened to me. I put off treatment because I was so terrified of it. Now I can say, "It's not that bad. It really isn't."

Anna
Food Demonstrator
Boca Raton, Florida

A Russian man, who works with my grandson claims that they make this tea in Russia and then they also eat the mushroom.

I don't know if it is mind over matter BUT I sure feel good since I'm drinking this tea drink. I feel so much stronger and my energy is coming back. I'm using this tea for approx. 4 months — I now walk 1 to 4 miles two and three times a week — don't feel dizzy any more. I'm 77 years young (every little bit helps). However, I am not on any medication — I hate to take medicine — don't want to fill my body with anything but food if possible.

Bret
Truck Driver
Mesa, Arizona

I have AIDS. In one month, my candida is gone, I'm gaining weight again, and I've been able to do yard work a couple hours a day. I wouldn't be surprised if my T-cells went up. I was almost bed ridden, now I'm running around everywhere, enjoying life again.

Joe
Retired salesman
Los Angeles, CA

In a couple of days, I had such energy — and I'm 71. I can do heavy work now if I want to, and I take care of things around the house, like paint and repair the roof. Dark hairs are starting to grow in my hair and mustache.

23

Anne
Former Nurse
Hollis, N.Y.

My blood pressure dropped. I had not been able to sit up in bed without grabbing the mattress and pull & push until I could sit up, with terrible pain. Now I can sit up with no trouble. I have back damage from an accident and arthritis. I dragged my left leg when I arise in the morning. Now I can pick it up.

Hemorrhoids were very painful before I started taking beverage. The pain subsided immediately. I've had no pain since. For some reason I was having headaches when I started taking beverage. Headaches left immediately. I am very heavy. I lost 18 lbs.

I had a lot of stress. Sometimes I felt like just collapsing. I no longer have stress. I am able to do more.

Leo
Bar Owner
Cedar Rapids, Iowa

I have shared the strange little things with a lot of people. I have noticed much success with them all. The greatest thing I have noticed is how it helps in digestion and also much improved skin.

A few months ago [my nutritionist] said, "Leo I saw this product at a conference. . . . It was like God taking me by the hand." She is a wonderful woman and I am sold on [the] mushroom.

James
Retired Airline Pilot
Irving, Texas

My wonderful M.D. recommended Kombucha because I have trouble with blood clots. Kombucha has heparin.

Mike
Consultant
Sierra Madre, CA

I have been using/drinking the Kombucha tea three weeks and my athlete's foot and acne [have] cleared up! My mom's arthritis is going away. Amazing stuff!

Dan
Senior Systems Analyst
South Bend, Indiana

I have been using Kombuchas for about 6 months now. I have had arthritis in my hands ... for about 36 years. I am 42 now!

I started noticing a relief from the arthritis, as well as a general feeling of well being after about a week. You get a lift from the tea as soon as you drink it the first time.

My hair is gradually losing its gray, as well as feeling thicker. My skin is not so sallow, I just look better. I also have lost about 12 pounds without trying. It has also helped to diminish my appetite, a pleasant side effect.

Neighborhood Interview

Kenneth Sikorsky shares experiences with Kombucha in the Berryville, Arkansas, neighborhood where he lives.

My neighbor's brother has cancer. He lost all his hair and was down to skin and bones. The doctors gave him 6 months to live. His mother got a tea mushroom from someone and he drank the tea for 6 months. Now he has gained 100 lbs and has a full head of hair. The doctors are growing [their] own tea mushroom trying to figure it out.

They gave me one mushroom. I'm 44 years old and have had 5 heart attacks around other health problems like fatigue, real bad indigestion, diabetes. For the last 10 years I have been spending most of my time on my back in bed unable to do much at all. After 3 days drinking the tea my indigestion [was] gone. I [had] to take 3 sleeping pills to get any sleep at all. [Then] I ran out of pills and started drinking the tea before I went to bed and I sleep like a baby. My chest pains are getting less and farther apart.

I've been being treated for depression for 10 years. With the tea I have such a sense of well being and a real peace of mind. I have been drinking 2 qts a day with no side effects at all.

Oh by the way I'm 6'3" and weigh 280 lbs and with the tea I have so much more energy I cleaned our whole house from top to bottom. This stuff is a Godsend!

I make 18 qts of this tea every 7 days. I have my wife drinking it and I have my 5 neighbors drinking it. I have not been selling it. I have been giving it to my Christian friends who need it.

Eric
Property Developer
Beverly Hills, CA

I have now been drinking . . . Kombucha tea for several months. I have prostate cancer and am a patient of an oncologist. . . I am on a combined hormone treatment and also have . . . tea three times daily. I told [my doctor] and he seemed quite interested and said, "By all means — go ahead with drinking this tea." I do believe it is beneficial.

I also have a hiatus hernia [which] causes me severe pain at times. Previously I found that a good tot of whiskey relieves the pain. But now I find that Kombucha tea can also stop this pain and obviously I now turn to this instead of relying on alcohol.

I start off every day with a small glass of Kombucha tea, without any sugar or anything, and I find it a great way to start the day.

William
Hair Stylist
Akron, Ohio

I can't say enough about the Kombucha tea, it's help[ed] me in many ways. My days are more productive. . . . I have scars on my face, it has taken the red out. I use it in [the] morning to freshen and tighten my adult face. I've lost 15 lb from the tea.

I use it (mushroom tea) in my hair as a rinse. It seems to have strengthen[ed] my hair; not so much hair is falling out. Plus I have friends that can't do without it now.

Peggy
Former Customer Service Manager
Seattle, Washington

*[My husband] is from Xian, which is the
ancient capital of China. . . . He's been watching me
. . . with the Kombucha and when he saw the first
one I made, he recognized it immediately. And he
said, "Oh yes, my family made these mushrooms.
And we drank the tea."*

*The first batch of tea I made was like nectar of
the gods. And he and I both just consumed it right
away.*

*In China the whole entire family lives together.
. . . He tells me this is something that went on in
their family. This was a family project.*

Terry
Film Production
Van Nuys, CA

Altho my last CD-4 T-cell count had jumped from 443 to 657, the next was 515—still not bad, and that reading happened during a minor sinus infection. Now it's in the upper 500's which is considered to be a high count.

I didn't go into this with the power of positive thinking. Sort of a doubting Thomas. When my T-cell count went up, I was stunned more than anything. I really couldn't attribute this to anything other than Kombucha.

Sally Ann
Bookseller
Culver City, CA

My tea mushrooms are getting bigger and look wonderful to me. The beverage itself has softened my skin and made it shine. My fingernails are stronger, my caffeine addiction has been transformed into enjoyment, not need. My appetite seems to be getting fine-tuned and I have an increased desire to drink pure, clean water.

I am just beginning to consume 12 ounces per day (tea beverage), so it will be interesting to see what the future produces for me in combo with the Kombucha. I do notice obviously a sense of gentleness and well being.

Alphonse
Retired
Perkasie, PA

My wife started on the Kombucha tea about three weeks ago. She is definitely more energized by the tea, and her diabetes daily testing shows an amazing decrease in her blood sugar content. I'm sure she will have to reduce her insulin strength or switch to oral medicine.

I too, have diabetes and am experiencing an improvement in my blood sugar and an increase of energy. I test my blood sugar once a day. I have a specialist who says an acceptable range is 70 to 140 if you can keep it there. I was ranging 135-170 over the last six months. I'm looking at a range now between 120-140. My wife's range used to be similar to mine, or higher. She's between 90-120.

Just the other day I took it over to a woman's house to show her how to use it. She had a group that meets regularly and asked me to talk to them. I sing in a barbershop quartet, and have since 1948. So I don't mind being in front of people.

We are harvesting four batches tomorrow (8 mushrooms coming out), with four new users.

<u>Adds wife Evelyn, "I haven't felt this well in twenty years."</u>

Lynda
Housewife
South Walpole, Mass

Lots of energy!

Pain in feet gone. Had it for months.

John
Recently Retired Teacher
New York, NY

General spirit, attitude and energy was very low. After one week of drinking the tea, all these improved. I have much more stamina.

Skin: itchy rash and scabbing. Improved a good bit after 2 weeks of the tea.

Jim
Social Worker
Los Angeles, CA

I have been suffering the pain of a hiatus hernia for about 15 years and was getting worse as the years went by. I have been drinking the Kombucha tea for two months. I have not had any pain since. I can eat anything I feel like, and I haven't been able to do that for many years. Prior to my knowledge of [the] tea, I was considering surgery.

Joe
Disabled
Cheyenne, Wyoming

I'm a male, 36 years old who is HIV+. For the months of Sept thru Nov 94 I had nausea which kept me from eating, resulting in a 35 lb weight loss. Although I had been receiving medication for the nausea it caused me to have diarrhea which also lasted well over two months.

Since drinking the Kombucha tea the cramping and diarrhea has stopped and I have gained fourteen or fifteen pounds back. My M.D. says that it is mostly likely the medications which are responsible for the improvements. But I know it's the tea.

Karen
Herbologist
Milwaukee, WI

I am up to 10 mushrooms now and very excited about the results.

My friend with MS has improved 75% since taking it. From [being] bed ridden to day time driving— she's come a long way.

I've had a slow, steady weight loss. Hurrah!

My 96 [year old] grandmother overcame pneumonia in just days.

Andrea
Registered Nurse
Newport Beach, CA

I started "brewing" the tea back in July. Post mastectomy — no problems thus far with any more cancer. I see my oncologist every 3 months and have lab work prior to each visit. So far, all of my lab values are excellent. So, I can at least attest to the tea's not causing me any harm. I do feel my complexion glows and a few people have said so as well.

The main thing I did notice was my craving for chocolate is virtually gone. I used to buy chocolate frequently when I would go grocery shopping. After drinking "the tea" I found myself in my old habit of looking at the chocolate bars at the store, but had no desire for them. So, I have gone months now without buying chocolate. I don't even look at it now!

I am a true believer in its healing and healthy properties and faithfully care for my "mushrooms" and drink my tea (and enjoy it immensely) every day.

Tom
Artist
Mesa, Arizona

I am living with AIDS. For the last four years I have been challenged with the most severe eosinophilic folliculitis, primarily on my arms and legs. Five dermatologists, "boo-coo" bucks, no relief. I started Kombucha in mid November.

Today, my arms are totally healed and the legs are coming along nicely. I'm so happy not to be covered with scabs and sores. It seems my mental health has also improved, a state of well being. My art has taken a playful attitude.

This is a magical gift from God and I treasure my "buchees." Not only surviving with AIDS — but thriving with AIDS.

Jane
Molecular Biologist
Chicago, Illinois

I have been brewing my batches for a month now. Things I have noticed are . . .

Much improved complexion! My chin is a trouble spot — oily and I get facial hairs I pluck out routinely. Well, this area is much less oily now, and I rarely pluck any hairs there any more. Isn't that odd. (And great!!)

I have recurrent interstitial cystitis. Since drinking Kombucha tea, my cystitis has calmed down to almost nothing! I read an article re: cystitis (the interstitial kind) in which heparin was used as part of the treatment and helped allay symptoms (pain, frequent need to urinate). I found it quite interesting that one component of Kombucha tea is heparin! I had been drinking cranberry juice or tea, and although it helped, the Kombucha tea seems to have done the trick! I have since taken to brewing the Kombucha tea (using green tea) and mixed it (after brewing) with brewed cranberry tea to which I also add raspberry tea bags: 3-4 cranberry tea bags and 2 raspberry. This makes an excellent and delicious drink. My boyfriend loves it!

It's going to be a lifetime drink for me.

Maureen
Office Administrator
Albuquerque, NM

I had been drinking the tea for five months when I went on vacation for two weeks. I didn't take my tea with me to drink and before I knew it I was sick with a cold. The first five months previous, I was never sick. I felt good and had lots of ambition.

I will never go without my tea again. A friend of mine made a batch for me before I got home so I could start taking it again right away.

Multiple Sclerosis Interview

Nancy Henshall is a remarkable woman who brightens the world around her despite, or perhaps because of, what she has seen in it.

I have MS — was diagnosed in April of '89. I went from using a cane — to a 4-prong cane — to a walker, which I am using now. I . . . had been unable to take regular steps with my walker, and HAD (past tense!) been bent over the walker, as I "scooted" along!

I began drinking my tea in the first week-and-a-half of December. By the time my son came home for the holidays, from Ft. Benning, Georgia, on the 17th of December, the exhaustion that came along with the MS was letting up on me. By Christmas Day, when we went to my cousins house — there was such a welcome change in my mobility!!! In her words, "You ran up the sidewalk!"

Of course I didn't literally run — but I was straight up, and taking step-after-step-after-step with my walker!! I am now doing so many things I have been unable to do for 1 - 2 years — and feel so much better than I have, in every bit that length of time!!

I have no other medication — or anything else that I take, other than the Kombucha tea I have been taking, that could account for my doing, and feeling, so very much better.

For every bit the length of time I mentioned, I have not been able to, myself alone, make dinner for my family, or make any "treats" for them because I couldn't get a cake batter from the mixing bowl to the pan. It sounds like such a simple thing — unless, after years of being a wife and mom who has always enjoyed doing this, and more, for my family, you all of a sudden can no longer do "the simple things."

What a thrill — no, what a true blessing, it is to be able to do these things again! I surprised my wonderful husband with, what to most, would be a simple batch of brownies. . . . The best part of the whole thing — I was able to do everything myself!! I was so happy to have a "Momma's Surprise" warm out of the oven for my husband — for the first time in years.

I can't tell you how much . . . regaining an ability that has been "lost" means to the person and their family — to actually be able to do things that you thought would never be a part of you again!

Tell us your experience with Kombucha—large or small—we want to know.

Write to: Kombucha
c/o Sierra Sunrise Books
14622 Ventura Blvd, Suite 800
Sherman Oaks, CA 91403

HOW TO MAKE KOMBUCHA TEA

If you decide to get a mushroom and make Kombucha tea, there are a few, easy steps you should follow.

People refer to this as the Betsy Pryor Method, but so far as we know, this is the only way to make the purest, most effective tea. It was created after searching through information and records that came from Europe and Asia where the tea has been made for many generations.

Some people suggest variations on this method, or say that certain precautions in handling the mushroom and tea are not necessary. For all we know, damaged mushrooms and weak tea may still produce some benefit. But to tell the truth, it hurts to even consider it.

Please. Start by doing it right. Completely right, as shown in the following pages. Get the full effect of Kombucha tea. After you see the results, we think you'll always want to do it this way.

BEFORE YOUR MUSHROOM ARRIVES

Once you've arranged to get a baby Kombucha mushroom from a friend or "grower" (see References section) you'll need to get a few things ready. It's like preparing for the arrival of another kind of baby. You're better off getting things ready before the event. (Good news: no diapers!)

HERE'S WHAT YOU'LL NEED

A 3- OR 4-QUART GLASS MIXING BOWL. The larger bowl is better to hold the full batch of tea you're going to make. The smaller bowl will work, but it's a very tight fit. Use clear, uncolored glass only. *No plastic, ceramic or crystal!* Later we'll explain how the tea may help to detoxify your body. For now, all you need to know is that it will try to detoxify the bowl. It'll pull out things like lead from crystal, cobalt from ceramics and petroleum by-products from plastic—and leave it in the tea. Who wants to drink that stuff? Plus it can get into the mushroom and stay for a long, long time. Use clear glass only! (Pyrex™ is good). Don't use a jar. Your Kombucha mushroom needs a large air surface for "breathing" space.

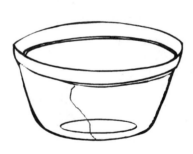

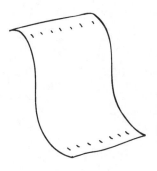

A WHITE BAKING TOWEL, FLOUR SACK CLOTH, or anything made of white, pure cotton and "breathable." An old, white, clean T-shirt, cut into a square will do. In fact, it helps to have two of them—so you can use one while the other's in the laundry. No cheesecloth, ever. It's much too porous and little fruit flies could get through. When you're ready to "harvest" your health beverage in a week or so, you can use the white cloth to strain the tea as you pour it through a **FUNNEL** into your refrigerator container. Then you can toss the old cloth in the wash and continue with the clean one.

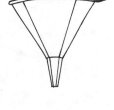

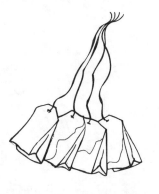

FOUR TEA BAGS of black tea (Lipton pekoe is okay).You can use three bags of green tea and one of black, if you prefer. (Some people believe green tea has anti-cancer properties.) Don't worry about the caffeine. There's almost none left at the end of the fermentation process. We'll talk about herbal teas later—they react in some good and not-so-good ways with the Kombucha. But while you're getting started, please stay with black or green tea.

49

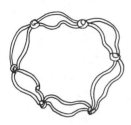

A LARGE, SIX-INCH RUBBER BAND. A piece of string *might* do. But we don't think you can get the tight fit with a string that keeps fruit or vinegar flies from crawling under the baking towel. If you don't have one, large rubber band, try tying several smaller ones end-to-end and make a circle big enough to stretch around the bowl.

A WOODEN OR PLASTIC SPOON. No metal should touch your mushroom! It tarnishes metal quickly, and that rusty stuff can get in the mushroom and tea. Ugh! Don't do it. Remember to remove rings and jewelry from your hands before 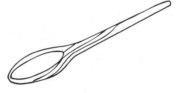 touching the mushroom. They're metal, right? (If you can't get a ring off, wear plastic gloves.)

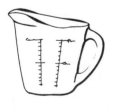

ONE CUP PURE WHITE CANE OR BEET SUGAR. Okay, okay. The stuff probably isn't healthy. Well, the mushroom eats it, not you, so just grit your teeth and pour. Besides, after a week to ten days, the sparkling health beverage you'll harvest has almost none of this sugar left.

Why not brown sugar? Russian scientists studying Kombucha found refined white sugar produced the best results. Brown sugar contains molasses and the mushroom can't digest it. Never use honey—it can kill or cripple the key bacteria in the Kombucha.

STAINLESS STEEL POT OR PAN, MINIMUM FOUR-QUART SIZE. We've used up to twenty-four-quart restaurant-quality stainless stock pots. (Bigger pots are great if you're making more than one batch of Kombucha.) You can use a metal pot because it won't come anywhere near the mushroom. But no aluminum! They get tarnished just sitting around in the kitchen. By the time you're ready to make tea, the stuff rubs off. Not good.

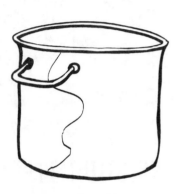

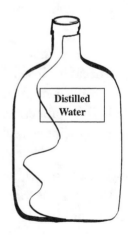

Distilled
Water

CLEAN, CLEAR WATER—3 quarts or more. If you're lucky enough to have pure well water where you live, no problem. The rest of us need to stop by the store and pick up some distilled water or use a water purifier. Just make sure there's no chlorine or other gunk in the water. And no water softeners.

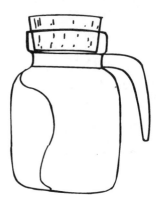

GLASS REFRIGERATOR CONTAINER to store the tea after your first "harvest." Each mushroom will produce about one or two quarts of tea, so plan ahead and get one or more containers. Clear glass only, and it's best if the container has a lid. Plastic lids are okay.

That's what you need. If you have these things on hand before the Kombucha arrives, you're all set to go!

SUBSTITUTIONS?

One rule. No ingredient or utensil substitutions. Ever. No matter what. Over the years, Kombucha has thrived where care was taken. It's also died out where not properly handled.

If you substitute honey, artificial sweetener or something else for sugar, or use herbal or decaf tea instead of black or green (the essential oils in some herbal or fruited tea can kill the mushroom), the healthy properties of the Kombucha tea are destroyed, and you might as well drink a soda pop.

Yes, yes, you say. The babies grown with substitute ingredients can look pretty good. But they're only ordinary yeast patties now, not true Kombucha.

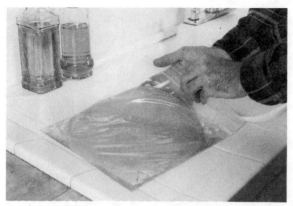

New mushroom arrives

THE FIRST TIME YOU MAKE TEA

You probably received your mushroom in an airtight plastic bag from a friend or distributor. Open the bag and let the mushroom breathe. Whew! It's going to smell "vinegary" but that's okay. Make sure you don't spill the tea inside, because you'll need it to "start" the fermenting process.

To keep your mushroom happy and healthy, don't let it come into contact with metal, direct sunlight or microwaves. Those things may cause it to break out in spots or even die. Much better to give it a little tender, loving care.

SO LET'S COOK!

Start by cleaning your hands, utensils, bowls and kitchen counter. Make sure dishes are out of the sink and there are no houseplants, fruit or open food containers around. The Kombucha has great defenses against mold spores and un-

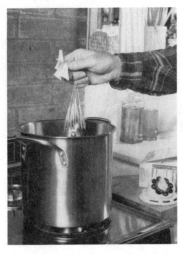

Boil water, add tea bags

friendly bacteria, but don't take chances. Keep things clean!

Bring 3 quarts of water to a boil (remember, distilled is best) in your stainless steel pot. Add 1 cup sugar and boil for another five minutes.

Turn off the heat, add four tea bags and let them steep for ten minutes. Remove the tea bags and let the brew cool a bit.

Ladle or pour the tea into your see-through glass mixing bowl. Let the tea cool to room temperature. Hot tea can damage the mushroom, so make sure it's cooled.

Add 6 ounces of the old tea at this point (if this is your first time, pour it from the plastic bag your mushroom came in.) Then gently place your Kombucha mushroom on top of the "growing tea." Let the darker, rougher side of the mushroom float face down in the new tea.

If needed, put two pieces of tape or some-

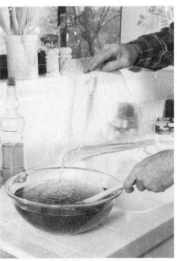

When new tea is cool, add old tea

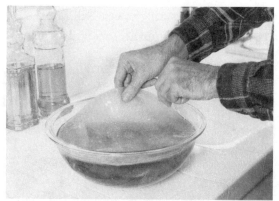

Place mushroom on tea

thing similar (no metal) across the top of the bowl. . . this keeps the white cloth from dipping into the tea. Cover with the cloth. Tie with string or pull the rubber band around the cloth to secure tea and mushroom against fruit flies, mold spores, etc. Place bowl in dim or dark, quiet, temperate, clean spot (about 70 to 90 °F) with adequate air-flow—such as a shelf in the kitchen, cellar, open closet, loft or attic. Not on the floor, if possible.

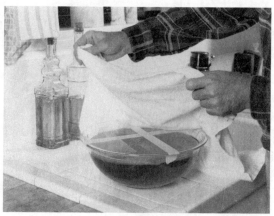

Cover with cloth

Remember, direct sunlight can kill your mushroom, so be careful. Also, the mushroom will give off a mild,

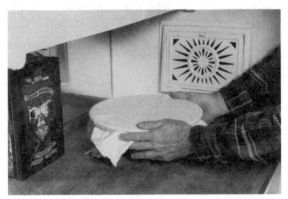

Put bowl in dim, quiet place

"vinegary" smell, so keep this in mind when choosing its new home. Don't move it around after the initial placement—that disturbs the fermenting process.

AFTER SEVEN TO TEN DAYS . . .

You're ready to harvest your new "baby" mushroom and refrigerate your sparkling health beverage! Remove the white cloth from your glass bowl. Notice that the "mother" mushroom (the one on bottom—the origi-

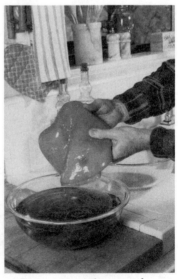

Remove mushrooms from bowl

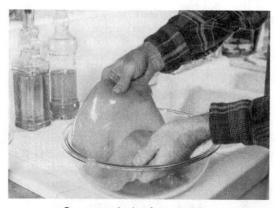

Separate baby from mother

nal one) has given birth to a baby (the one on top). Make sure your hands are clean and take off any jewelry (no metal, remember?). Remove both mushrooms from the bowl (they might be stuck together) and separate baby from mother by pulling apart gently.

Put them in another glass bowl or deep dish with just enough newly harvested tea to cover them.

Now pour the newly fermented Kombucha tea from the glass bowl (using the white cloth as a strainer) into a clear glass container (the funnel is a big help here) and place your tea in the refrigerator. All right! Chill, and it's ready to drink.

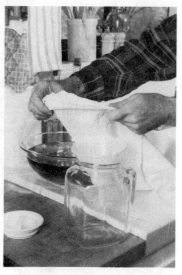

Prepare to pour tea...with funnel and white cloth

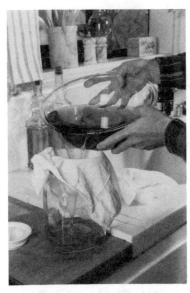

Pour through the cloth

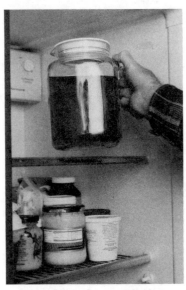

Store tea in refrigerator

We'll tell you more about storing and using the tea later.

NOW, START AGAIN RIGHT AWAY

Don't let mushrooms sit on the counter for more than 30 minutes. Leaving them out longer can attract mold or fruit flies and weaken the culture. And *never* put them in plastic bags to store in the refrigerator. This can cause toxic reactions and cripple the mushroom.

Brew a fresh batch of "growing tea" using the two mushrooms. You can double the amount of tea you make by putting each mushroom in a separate bowl. Just double the recipe (water, tea, sugar) and follow the same steps.

HOW MANY MUSHROOMS WILL YOU WANT TO KEEP?

That depends. We've discovered that after seven to ten days of fermenting, a 3-quart bowl will yield about 1 1/2 quarts of Kombucha tea. If you drink the recommended 12 ounces a day (that's 84 ounces a week or about 2 1/2 quarts) you'd need to ferment two mushrooms per week per person. In Eastern Europe and Asia, families grow their mushrooms in larger bowls. You can do this, too. Simply adjust the recipe to reflect the number of quarts in the larger bowl.

Always remember that the mushroom needs a large surface to "breathe." So no "sun tea" jars, small-mouthed containers or fish bowls. Don't worry if the larger surface area is bigger than your mushroom. When you make the first batch of tea, the "mom" will make a "baby" mushroom that exactly fits the new, larger container!

PROBLEMS THAT MAY COME UP AND WHAT TO DO ABOUT THEM

BUBBLES

The Kombucha mushroom is kind of ugly in a cute sort of way. Don't worry if it gets little bubbles or "warts." These are usually on the side that faces down in the "growing tea," and are simply air pockets. Gently press the bubble out with your hands.

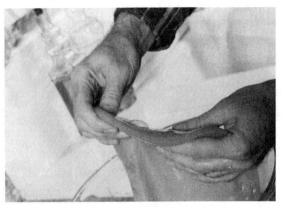

"Air bubble"

HOLES

The side that faces up is usually shiny, smooth, and lighter in color, but not always perfect. If holes form when you separate the mom from the baby, don't worry. Your Kombucha will still make a terrific tea.

MOLD

If for some reason you get mold on your mushroom (we've never seen this, but they say it can happen) older sources say to just remove it by dunking the mushroom in a bowl of vinegar for a few minutes, then rinsing under the tap. But...we recommend starting with a fresh mushroom and not drinking or using that tea as "starter." Some molds have no effect. Others could be very harmful.

To avoid getting mold in the first place, follow the easy instructions in this book. Normally, you won't ever get mold unless something isn't done right. That's because the

Kombucha tea is slightly acidic, and eliminates most germs that come near it. It also has a mild anti-bacterial ingredient that gives added protection.

Kombucha tea is protected better than most of the food in your kitchen. How can you help the Kombucha protect itself? Don't leave the mushroom exposed to air for a long time during "harvest." Always add 6 ounces of old tea to the new batch. Don't put your Kombucha near any plants. Keep it covered with a cloth while it's growing. Keep the tea in a covered container in the refrigerator after harvest.

SHRED

If the mushroom looks a little "worse for wear" after harvesting, rinse it under the tap in lukewarm water (unless you have heavily chlorinated water—then dip in distilled water or use a water purifier). This will clear off the harmless, little brown culture "tags."

TOO HOT

Putting the mushroom into new tea that is too hot (over 100°F) can cripple or kill it. Always let new tea cool to room temperature before adding the mushroom or the 6 ounces of old tea.

If your mushroom drops to the bottom of the bowl, it usually means the tea has not cooled enough. Unless the tea was *very* hot, your mushroom is still okay. Don't worry about it.

WORN

If the mushroom turns really brown, it might be old and tired. Discard (bury it in a garden or whatever) and continue with the "baby." If treated with love and kindness, the offspring of your mushroom should last a lifetime.

CROWDED

You shouldn't put more than one mushroom into a batch of tea. Believe it or not, some people don't remove the "babies," and let the mushroom get very, very thick. This will cause some of the mushrooms to starve—there's not enough nutrients in a batch of tea for all of them. Use one mushroom in each bowl of tea, and give the others away.

THIN

If your baby mushroom is thin and scrawny when you harvest it, that usually means it was too cold. Try to keep the temperature between 70 to 90 °F. In winter, it may help if you put more than 6 ounces of harvested tea into the bowl of new tea before adding the mushroom—this helps jump-start the process. If the temperature falls below 70 degrees while it's brewing, give the mushroom two or three more days to grow. If it was not too cold, maybe something is vibrating near it, like a refrigerator, microwave, washing machine or car. By the way, they don't seem to do well with cigarette smoke around them.

VACATION

If you need to leave the mushroom alone for a month or two, float it in a 3-4 quart or larger clear glass bowl of "growing tea," covered with flour sack towel and a rubber band. Place it in a cool, dark spot—your refrigerator will do—at about 42 to 48 °F. When you return, throw out the old tea and make a fresh batch the normal way. Then start the harvest cycle again. It should be fine.

FREEZING

Never freeze your Kombucha. That only works in an industrial, quick-freeze unit. In a slow-freeze refrigerator (like you have at home) crystallization of cells can occur, causing them to burst and cripple or kill the mushroom. If you're not going to use the Kombucha for a long time, give it to a friend or neighbor. They'll return the favor some day.

REPLACEMENT

That brings up something very important. Lots of times you hear people talking about using extraordinary methods to repair a Kombucha when it's been damaged. They try to cut out a piece of mold, or "breed out" contaminants caused by growing it in plastic. Don't do it.

One of the great things about Kombucha is that when you make a batch of tea, you get a free "baby" mushroom. You can use the first few mushrooms yourself, but will soon find you're up to your whatever in extra mushrooms. Give them to relatives, friends or people down the street. Let them share some of the good feelings you get from staying healthy.

And, let those people be your back-up in case your mushroom gets scalded or you go on a long vacation.

You'll find they're more than happy to give you their next "baby"—clean, fresh and healthy.

HOW TO GIVE SOMEONE A KOMBUCHA

Once people experience the good health and good feelings that come with Kombucha, they often get excited about sharing it with other people. The great part is... you get a free mushroom after every harvest. You *can* share it—with friends, people at work or people you meet at social events. Here's how.

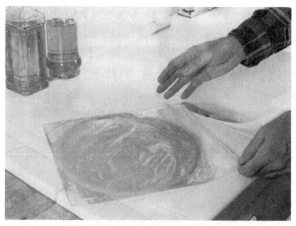

Give baby mushroom a friend

First and most important, raise your mushroom well. Keep your own Kombucha mushroom well-cared-for and it will produce beautiful "babies."

If you tell people about your Kombucha experiences and they ask for a mushroom, agree to let them have your next "baby" (some people actually have a waiting list of relatives and neighbors). Don't stack your extra mushrooms in the refrigerator or freeze them like fish fillets—it can severely damage them. At the very least, it will reduce their ability to make tea for a while, and the person receiving your gift will probably assume (correctly) something is wrong. Give them a good experience. Give them only a fresh mushroom, directly from your harvest.

While they're waiting a few days for the fresh mushroom, you should advise them to get ready. They'll need to pick up things like a clear glass bowl, tea, sugar, and the other items listed in this book. To help, you should copy a set of instructions for them so they know what to expect and what to do. If you really care about them, you could give a copy of this book—or send them down to the bookstore to get their own.

When harvest day comes, you should have a plastic freezer-quality bag on hand. When you separate the baby mushroom from the mother, place the new mushroom in the bag and add 6 ounces of newly harvested tea. Then press the side of the bag gently to remove most of the air from it, and seal the top tightly.

Place the bag out of the sunlight and not near a microwave. It would be great, of course, if the person receiving the mushroom was standing right there and could run home with it to start their own tea. That rarely happens. But it should get into their hands as soon as possible, and they should get the mushroom into it's own bowl of tea within a few days—seven days at the most.

The fun part comes a couple weeks later—when they've had time to make some tea and drink it for a while. You know that time has come when you see the smile on their face. The hard part is... you then have to listen to *their* great experiences. Oh, well.

HERBAL TEA

The good news about herbal tea is that it can give a different (some people say "much better") taste to the Kombucha tea. Herbal teas may also add beneficial vitamins and other good things.

The bad news is that using herbal tea to grow Kombucha may damage the Kombucha and drastically weaken the benefits of the tea. This happens because many herbs contain what is called volatile oil, and a high dose of it is harmful to the Kombucha.

Several references show the amount of these volatile oils in herbs, and that can guide you if you're serious about finding a way to include herbs in your Kombucha tea. Unfortunately, different references give different answers. Some recommend chamomile, others say "never!"

We recommend you brew healthy, herbal tea by itself and enjoy it—but not use herbal tea to *make* Kombucha.

Also, some people ask if they can heat Kombucha like other teas before drinking it. Don't! Kombucha tea contains organic fluids that can be destroyed by heat.

(For more about what's in Kombucha, see the "History and Research" section.)

WHEN YOU GET A NEW MUSHROOM

Is it healthy and well-grown? How do you know? Look at it—is there any mold? Politely ask the person giving it to you how it was raised. Did they use clean and careful methods like the ones described here? How long has it been out of its bowl of tea, sitting in a plastic bag? Seven days is the longest it can go before beginning to starve.

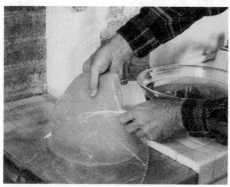

Check new mushroom carefully

Be aware—a damaged mushroom will not give you good tea. And if it's moldy it can be dangerous. Be safe. Use a healthy mushroom.

MAKE A FRIEND

No time to raise a Kombucha while you race around in your hectic life? Is your house or apartment too small to give the Kombucha bowls their own growing space?

Find a friend in the neighborhood to make the tea for you. There's almost always someone in the neighborhood who's retired, a homemaker, or has a disability that keeps them close to home. Work out a trade. They may need help with a chore around the house or some other compensation. In return, they can give you a ready supply of Kombucha tea.

Actually, once a person is making tea for themselves, there's very little work in filling a few additional bowls for neighbors. And there's a tremendous payback—people who receive the tea tend to be very grateful and in good spirits. It's a rewarding experience.

If you're the one receiving the tea, remember a little appreciation goes a long way.

SUMMARY

The next two pages contain an easy-to-read visual summary of the "Betsy Pryor Method." Use it in combination with the detailed discussions on the previous pages.

THE BETSY PRYOR METHOD

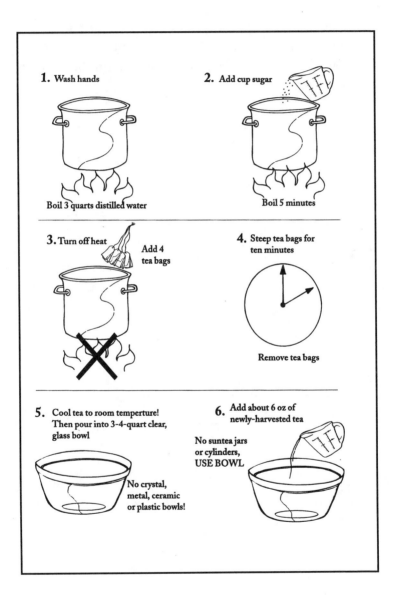

1. Wash hands

Boil 3 quarts distilled water

2. Add cup sugar

Boil 5 minutes

3. Turn off heat

Add 4 tea bags

4. Steep tea bags for ten minutes

Remove tea bags

5. Cool tea to room temperture! Then pour into 3-4-quart clear, glass bowl

No crystal, metal, ceramic or plastic bowls!

6. Add about 6 oz of newly-harvested tea

No suntea jars or cylinders, USE BOWL

FOR KOMBUCHA TEA

7. Float mushroom on top of tea--
rougher, darker side down

NO metal
should touch
mushroom

Room temperature

8. Put tape across top of bowl
(optional)

Cover with thin, freshly laundered
white cloth, and rubberband

9.

Place in a dim, clean,
quiet, ventilated space,
7-10 days, 70-90 degrees.

10. Then remove mushrooms,
gently separate.

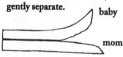

baby

mom

Start over right away. Don't
store in plastic bags in refrigerater
or leave out in open.

11.

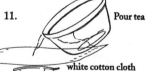

Pour tea

white cotton cloth

funnel

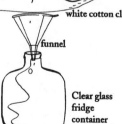

Clear glass
fridge
container

12.

Drink 4 ounces three times
a day--before, after or between
meals. Whenever!
To your health!

DRINKING THE TEA AND OTHER USES

The Kombucha health beverage tastes like a light Moselle wine or a really snappy apple cider. Normally, you drink 4 ounces on an empty stomach before breakfast. This gives you a terrific energy boost — a great way to start the day! Later drink another 4 ounces before lunch and dinner if you want to lose weight. Or, if you're happy with your weight and want to help your digestive process, drink 4 ounces after lunch and dinner or any time in between.

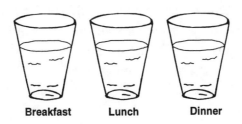

Breakfast **Lunch** **Dinner**

A real life experience: "Without changing my eating habits, I lost 14 pounds in a few months, and gained a wonderful feeling of renewed well-being and energy within the first week."

Everyone is built differently, but feeling better and having much more energy is described by many people.

Sometimes people drink more or less than 12 ounces a day. Let your body tell you.

If the refrigerated health beverage seems a little too strong for your taste, add an ounce of distilled water to your 4 ounce drink. Some people mix juices with the tea to give some variety to the taste, but it's possible that strong juices can interfere with the healthful qualities of the tea. If you really want a good, healthy result, only mix with water. If you're basically healthy and are just using this for a tune-up, go ahead and experiment.

But — never mix something with Kombucha tea and let it sit in the refrigerator or on the counter. The tea continues to "grow" slightly, even in the fridge. Putting something else in it can weaken the tea and possibly cause an unpleasant reaction. If you really want to use a mixture, do it in the glass just before you drink it.

Another way to adjust the tea to suit your taste is to make the fermenting time a little shorter or longer. A lot will depend on your climate, altitude, season of the year and even phase of the moon. Experiment. We've heard that brewing the tea for much less time (2 to 5 days) produces a sweeter taste but may reduce the benefits tremendously.

On the other hand, if you feel the tea is giving you some real health benefits and you want to get the most out of it, let the tea "grow" longer — ten to fourteen days. This makes the tea stronger, and also gives it a more "tart" flavor. It definitely packs a wallop.

DRINKING TEA THE FIRST TIME

Kombucha tea has its own natural flavor—which is reasonable considering it's extraordinary effect.

If you're a first-time drinker, or giving it to someone who is, there are a couple things you should know.

The tea is always sweetest right after harvest. It tastes like carbonated apple cider. After that, the tea continues to "grow" slowly. By the end of the week, just before you make your next harvest, you'll notice the old tea tastes much stronger and a bit more "sharp."

Do first-time drinkers a favor: give them newly harvested tea.

Some people compare Kombucha to drinking coffee. The first time most people try coffee, they wonder why it's so popular. After a while they find themselves at the local cafe paying extra to get the strong stuff.

When drinking Kombucha tea, quantity is also important. Don't overdo it at first. We recommend only drinking 2 ounces three times a day during the first week. By strange and wonderful coincidence, that's exactly how much tea is made by one mushroom.

At the first harvest, when you separate the "baby" mushroom from the "mother," you can make two bowls of tea the second week. That should produce enough for you to drink 4 ounces each time from then on.

STORING YOUR TEA

You'd be surprised. No matter how often it's mentioned, someone will store their tea in a plastic container. Please

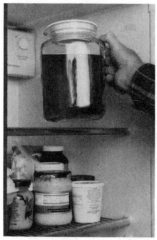

don't! As we pointed out before, the tea could draw out petroleum by-products, and you don't want to drink that!

Use clear glass containers only. And keep it refrigerated or cooled. You know by now that the tea continues to "grow" even after the mushroom is removed. Without refrigeration it may get sour before you have a chance to drink it.

Store in glass container in refrigerator

If the tea has to sit out for some reason, shake it occasionally to keep a new mushroom from trying to form on top of it.

Even in the fridge, you'll notice some stuff settles to the bottom of the container. These are little bits of healthy yeast and shreds of mushroom. This is normal, and you'll tend to get more of it as the week goes on. Some people eat the little pieces of mushroom and swear it improves their digestion. Some people leave it in the bottom of the jar and wash it out at the end of the week. It's up to you.

The tea shouldn't be kept in storage longer than four weeks after it's been made. Old studies indicate that if

Kombucha is bottled, it can keep for up to five months. But not when sitting in a container in your refrigerator. To be on the safe side, we recommend you toss the old tea and make a fresh batch.

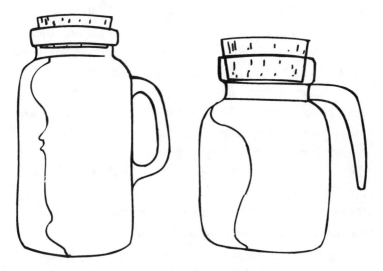

You can store the tea in any size bottle but, remember, the bottle must be clear glass

Some enterprising people noticed that if the tea gets very old, it can taste like vinegar. So they actually use it for that purpose and sprinkle it over salads as a healthy substitute. Do whatever works for you.

KOMBUCHA TEA IN HEALTH FOOD STORES

Finding bottled Kombucha in stores is becoming more common now. It saves people the work of "growing" it themselves. On the other hand, it's not cheap (about

$5.00 per pint at places we visited) and the quality of the tea can vary widely.

We've never bottled it, since it's always available fresh. But we did talk to people at health food stores, bought some bottled tea and tried it. Here are some thoughts.

The cleanliness and care of the person making the tea are not apparent by looking at the bottle, so you should be careful to buy it from a reputable store. The benefit you get from the tea will also depend on how long it was "grown." You have to hope for the normal seven to ten day period. Some producers might grow it for only two to three days so they can make more bottles of tea every week—good for them, but not so good for you. There could be little or no benefit from young tea. A short growing time and long "bottled" time might offset each other, or might not. Ask questions and use your judgment.

The taste of the beverage will change depending on how long it sits in the bottle, since it continues to ferment. An old bottle may taste somewhat sour.

Some bottlers also mix herbs, honey and other ingredients with the Kombucha. Check the label, and see if this is something you want.

If you decide to use store-bought Kombucha, reach for glass bottles only. No plastic.

OTHER USES

Though the main use for Kombucha is as a healthy beverage, people have found other good ways to use the tea and the mushroom—as a facial tonic, for example.

From a woman in Los Angeles: "I got the idea after the Northridge earthquake. After a week of living on a closed mountain road that looked like it had been hit by a bomb, my skin was a wreck! The stress of all the quake damage and aftershocks had aged it ten years. The Kombucha restored it to normalcy within a few days, and now my friends are telling me that my skin never looked better."

For cold sores and skin eruptions, several people have mentioned that a piece of mushroom can be applied directly to the area affected. Moving a little further afield, an exotic dancer said it helped clear up her herpes in a couple of days.

Directly applying the mushroom has apparently also helped with burns. Jenny, a set painter in Hollywood, got a bad sunburn and put her mushroom on the worst area. The next morning, there was a tan circle where the mushroom had been. The rest was still red and painful.

Gargling with the tea has also been found to help with sore throat or gum infections.

Many people report benefits for pets and other animals similar to what people experience. Dogs and cats need only four to eight eyedroppers-full of tea in their water dish each day. Among aging dogs and cats the results are especially visible. These include improvements in their hair, hearing, eyesight and temperament.

During flea season, their skin can be soothed by mixing equal amounts of tea and water. Spray it on flea-irritated areas or apply it directly to the hot spot with a cotton ball.

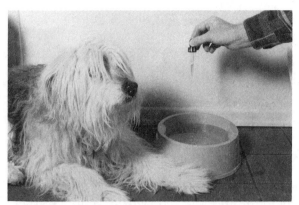

Four to eight drops can benefit your pets

For horses, up to a gallon of tea can be put into a standard trough filled with water. People also report giving tea to ostriches, dairy cows and other animals, but we don't have information on how much tea was used.

SIDE EFFECTS?

So far the tea has been used for many generations, and the only "side effect" mentioned from time to time is some nausea if a person drinks too much tea too quickly.

A doctor in Santa Monica had an experience with that. Several patients told him they use Kombucha, so he has had a chance to learn their experiences. One patient reported feeling nauseous so he recommended she stop for a few days. She did, then started again and felt fine.

Other side effects? Many studies have been done in Europe and Russia over the last hundred years (see

References) and several times they said conclusively, "no side effects."

HOW DO YOU FEEL?

You should always feel the same or better after drinking Kombucha tea.

If something unusual happens and you feel worse, stop taking it while you check out the following possibilities.

If you're taking medications and drinking the tea, there is a possibility that might cause upset. We haven't heard reports of bad combinations, but play it safe. Consult your health care provider.

If one or more of the "clean and careful" handling methods for making and storing the tea have not been followed and the mushroom has become crippled or contaminated, you could have a physical reaction. If this happens, don't fool around. Throw away the mushroom and the tea made from it. Get a clean, healthy mushroom and start again.

And check every step. Somewhere along the line you'll find someone took a shortcut and put the mushroom in boiling tea, used a plastic container or something else. **No shortcuts.**

HISTORY AND RESEARCH

CHINA

It is widely believed that as early as 220 BC in China—during the Tsin dynasty—people tried to find immortality through the use of fungus treatments, which they believed had magical properties. There was one variety prized above all others, known to the Chinese as Ling-tche, the Divine Tea. This is the unique combination of natural ingredients that has come down to us through the generations as Kombucha.

Today there is something marketed in China as "Ling-tche" which we are told is not Kombucha. If you happen to be shopping there, be careful.

JAPAN

In 414 AD, the Japanese Emperor Inkyo was reported to be suffering from severe digestive troubles, and summoned a physician from Korea. This doctor Kombu is believed to have brought the divine tea to Japan. (Kombu is also the name of a Japanese brown seaweed, so watch what you get there.)

In later years, Japanese warriors considered the properties of this divine tea so special that they carried it into battle in their field flasks. This is believed to be one of the few times the tea was fermented on the move. Historical archives indicate that their habit was to top off the ferment in their hip flasks with fresh tea, allowing some of the old culture to ferment the new tea. They considered it a refreshing and strengthening beverage.

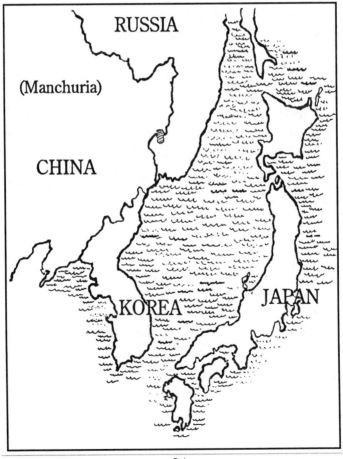

RUSSIA

Historians indicate that as trade routes extended, oriental merchants probably carried the mushroom with them to Russia. From there it made its way into Eastern Europe. The habit of drinking this fermented tea then became quite acceptable throughout Europe.

It is common to see stories of grandmothers tending a pot of Kombucha in the corner of small, rustic homes and doling it out to family members stricken by illnesses or other maladies.

One of the many local names given to Kombucha over the years grew out of this experience. A woman traveling in Russia saw that many villagers in Kargasok lived to ripe old ages in good health and she searched for their "secret." It turned out that each hut had one or more pots of this amazing tea brewing, and the tea was given to all members of the family as a normal part of their life. Reports of this miraculous "Kargasok tea" spread the use of Kombucha even farther.

EUROPE

As Kombucha was passed from family to family across Europe in the late 1800's, it attracted the interest of health professionals. German doctors and scientists studied the Kombucha mushroom and tea in great detail from 1900 until World War II. During the war, strict rationing and widespread shortage of two essential ingredients, tea and

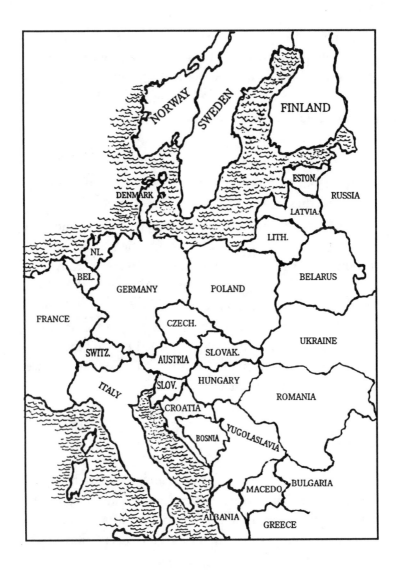

sugar, almost wiped out the use of Kombucha in Europe, including much of Russia.

Fortunately, some of the mushrooms were preserved and a resurgence of Kombucha began after the war. Italian high society, for example seemed to have had a real passion for this fermented tea during the 1950's.

As an interesting footnote, **Günther Frank** reports that in 1952 **Stalin's** personal physician (Vinogradov), aware of Stalin's fear of cancer, ordered tests on Kombucha, which was believed to help prevent it. Satisfied that Kombucha at least had no bad effects, the doctor gave this tea to the Soviet leader. Unfortunately, two KGB officers (Ryumin and Ignatiev) tried to improve their position with Stalin by claiming he was being poisoned. The doctor was jailed and rumors quickly spread that this drink (which Russians call "tea kvass") was likely to produce cancer. Use of the tea plummeted. When Stalin died in 1953, the KGB officers were put in jail and the doctor was vindicated. A book published in Russia by Barbancik in 1954 dispelled the rumor.

A few years later in the 1960's scientific research in Switzerland found that drinking Kombucha was at least as beneficial as eating yogurt. It's popularity soon increased and it became widely available again.

One of the people credited with extensive research into the properties and beneficial use of Kombucha is **Dr. Rudolf Sklenar** in Germany. He used it in his medical practice and gave the mushrooms to his patients from about 1951 until his death in 1987. He reported that "Kombucha produced good therapeutical results in cases of metabolic diseases, also with those of a chronical nature... In no instance undesired side or late effects caused by a treatment with these therapeutics were ascertainable." He recommended it as one of the beneficial treatments for people suffering from cancer.

Today, the two recognized authorities on Kombucha in Europe are Dr. Sklenar's niece and collaborator, **Rosina Fasching** in Austria, and Günther Frank in Germany.

UNITED STATES

The Kombucha mushroom came to America on a significant scale in 1993 when **Betsy Pryor** obtained a Kombucha mushroom indirectly from Manchuria by way of Sister Joan Derry of the Brahma Kumaris Center. When Ms. Pryor gave baby mushrooms to her older neighbors, the quiet canyon street soon became active with people tending their gardens and showing more energy than they had in years. She gave other mushrooms to people in the AIDS community and saw similar effects. Based on those positive experiences, she began to distribute this productive strain of Kombucha across the country.

Over the past couple of years, she has grown and sent out more than 10,000 mushrooms, and each of them has been doubling every seven to ten days. Even if we assume two-thirds of all new mushrooms are discarded or used for something other than making tea, the descendants of her mushrooms probably number over two million in the United States today.

The Kombucha mushroom and tea are now available in all fifty states.

Prof. Eduard Stadelmann at the University of Minnesota has researched Kombucha for over fifty years. From 1957 to 1961, while teaching at Univerisität Freiburg in Switzerland, he published several widely-quoted articles which surveyed the field of research into Kombucha, and included over 200 references.

Stadelmann began using Kombucha in Europe in 1930, and is very familiar with the people who have studied it. In 1960 he sent a mushroom to **Clifford Hessletine**, President of the Mycological Society of America, whose laboratory tests confirmed the tea produced antibacterial activity. The results were published in 1965.

Stadelmann keeps track of progress being made on Kombucha studies in Europe, and keeps in touch with people in the United States and around the world who work with it.

Dr. Jeffrey Gates and **Dr. Keith Steinkraus** at Cornell University are actively involved in the search for better understanding of the medical effects of Kombucha.

Dr. Steinkraus is a recognized expert in the field of fermentation, and has personally used Kombucha for ten years.

Dr. Gates has worked with Kombucha for the past year, and is particularly interested in it as a possible treatment for gastrointestinal disorders (ulcers, etc.) as well as examining its possible effect on tumors, cancer prevention, prostate and breast cancer.

We hope foundations and other institutions will provide the financial support to continue this good work.

Drs. Richard and **Rachael Heller** are very interested in Kombucha because it may be related to other work they have been doing. They are professors at Mount Sinai School of Medicine in New York, and the best-selling authors of *Healthy for Life*.

"A ROSE BY ANY OTHER NAME . . ."

As you might expect from something that has become established in many countries over hundreds of years, Kombucha is known by many names. These are some of the ones you may see when books or articles are translated into English from another language.

NAMES FOR THE MUSHROOM

Brinum-Ssene (Latvian)
Cainii grib (Russian)
Cainogo griba (Georgian)
Chamboucho (Romanian)
Champignon de longue vie (French)
Combucha (Japanese)
Fungus japonicus (Pharmaceutical name)
Funko cinese (Italian)
Hongo (Spanish)
Japán gomba (Hungarian)
Kargasok-Teepilz (German)

Kombucha (International usage)
Olinka (Bohemian and Moravian
   monasteries)
Tea mould (Java)
Teepilz (German)
Teyi saki (Armenian)
Theezwam Komboecha (Dutch)

NAMES FOR THE BEVERAGE

Cainii kvass (Russian)
   This is usually translated
   "tea kvass." Do not confuse it
   with "kvass," the Russian name
   for a sour beer.
Cainogo kvassa (Georgian)
Elixir de longue vie (French)
Kombucha tea (English)
Kombucha-thee (Dutch)
Kombuchagetränk (German)

Sometimes people talk about different parts of the Kombucha mushroom or tea, particularly in scientific studies. In those cases, you may see references to names in the next section.

TECHNICAL STUFF

Technically speaking, Kombucha is not a mushroom or fungus. It's a symbiosis (beneficial combination) of healthy bacteria and yeast. The Moscow Central Bacteriological Institute states that it's formed from Bacterium xylinum and nest-like deposits of yeast cells of the genus Saccharomyces. This mixture includes: Saccharomyces ludwigii, Saccharomyces of the apiculatus types, Bacterium xylinoides, Bacterium gluconicum, Schizosaccharomyces pombe, Acetobacter ketogenum, Torula types, Pichia fermentans and other yeasts

They also say that a key ingredient of the Kombucha tea is glucuronic acid, which binds up poisons and toxins, both the environmental and metabolic kind, and flushes them out of the body via the kidneys. This is a natural body function which your liver and kidneys do every day, by producing their own glucuronic acid. The tea simply boosts this normal process.

Glucuronic acid is also a building block of a group of important polysaccharides in the body, including hyaluronic acid (a basic component of connective tissue), chondroitin sulfate (a basic component of cartilage), mucoitinsulfuric acid (a building block of the stomach lining and the vitreous humor of the eye), and heparin.

A very small amount of alcohol is produced (.5%, the same as "non-alcoholic beer") and the Kombucha tea is lightly carbonated.

The beverage also contains Vitamins B_1, B_2, B_3, B_6, B_{12}, as well as folic acid and L-lactic acid, a substance rarely present in the connective tissue of cancer patients, the lack of which is believed to result in failure of cell respiration and the build-up of undesirable DL-lactic acid in the tissues. Kombucha tea also contains usnic acid which has an antibacterial effect.

THEORIES

What happens when people drink Kombucha tea is usually described as one—or a combination—of the following:

DIGESTION involves stomach acid dissolving food and making it ready to be absorbed into the body. Kombucha is somewhat acidic and may help this process, without being so strong as to cause an upset stomach. The tea also contains "people friendly" bacteria which may work with the body's natural bacteria to help finish the digestion process. Dr. Jim Blechman in Southern California suggests better digestion could explain people's claims of increased energy, regularity, and improved skin with fewer wrinkles.

But he is far from the first to point out improvement of digestion. In 1928 Dr. Mollenda in Germany reported, "In the case of angina, especially when there is a coating of the tonsils, the drink should not merely be used for gargling but for drinking, and that for the destruction of bacteria which reach the stomach through food and drink. . . . Even though the beverage is acidic, it does not cause any acidic condition in the stomach; it facilitates and noticeably promotes the digestion even of difficult to digest foods. Equally favorable successes after taking Kombucha beverage have also been reached for gouty eczema and for stones in kidneys, urine and gall."

TOXINS are normally removed from the body by the liver and kidneys using glucuronic acid. As we mentioned, this acid binds itself to toxins and allows them to be removed from the body as waste. Since glucuronic acid has been identified in Kombucha tea, the additional supply may allow the body to remove more toxins, which in turn allows the body to function in the normal, natural way it did before toxins built up.

If this is of interest to you, check the books in our reference section by **Artz** and **Osman** (1950) and **Dutton** (1966 and 1980). They follow glucuronic acid from its discovery in 1879 through all the steps of analysis on how detoxification works in the body, drawing on research by experts from many countries.

ANTIBACTERIAL properties of the Kombucha tea have been well documented in studies in the United States (see Hesseltine), Germany and Russia. This might explain the generations-old tradition of grandmothers giving it to family members who suffer from a variety of illnesses.

VITAMINS present in the tea may also contribute to the feeling of general well-being identified by people who use Kombucha.

What is the real answer? Only additional controlled, scientific tests will tell. We hope American universities will take on this challenge. It would be good to know the answer.

REFERENCES

WHERE TO FIND A KOMBUCHA MUSHROOM

There are many places you can get Kombucha mushrooms across the United States. If you ask people where you work or put a message on the local market bulletin board, you're likely to find someone who can give you one. Anybody with a Kombucha gets a "baby" mushroom every week or ten days and is usually happy to share with someone who's interested.

Normally they'll insist you have it free. You often find that people who use Kombucha feel a small miracle fell into their life, and are happy to share their experience.

If for some reason that route doesn't get you a mushroom, you can contact one of the commercial growers across the country.

Betsy Pryor, in addition to appearing on television and radio, and speaking to live groups about Kombucha, is the founder of Laurel Farms™, widely recognized as the leader among American growers. They charge a fee for their mushrooms, but make special arrangements for people suffering from serious illnesses who cannot afford the normal fee.

Whether your mushroom comes from a friend or a grower, try to learn if they follow the clean "growing" method described in this book. You need a healthy mushroom to get good results.

INFORMATION

For further information or to obtain a Kombucha mushroom, send a stamped, self-addressed envelope to:

> Ms. Betsy Pryor
> Laurel Farms
> P.O. Box 7405
> Studio City, California 91614

Here are two other reliable sources of information on the Kombucha mushroom. Be sure to enclose a self-addressed envelope and international postage voucher for reply.

> Mr. Günther Frank
> Genossenschafts Strasse 10
> 75217 Birkenfeld im Schwartzwald
> Germany

> Ms. Rosina Fasching
> Post Box 98
> A-9021 Klagenfurt
> Austria

INTERNET

Another outstanding source is the **Internet**, if you're interested in cyber-talking with people who know about

Kombucha. As a good starting place, we recommend the Kombucha Tea Cider Gopher sponsored by Arizona State University at:

enuxsa.eas.asu.edu 6600

On **Prodigy**, access the Health Bulletin Board. We saw a lively discussion there in the topic area of Holistic Medicine and the specific subject of Kombucha.

America-On-Line has a bulletin board (or "forum") called Longevity which had a good discussion on Kombucha. Some of the individuals kept in touch afterward and exchanged personal e-mail and experiences with Kombucha.

BOOKS AND ARTICLES

Abele, Johann (In German): Teepilz Kombucha bei Diabetes? Der Naturarzt. vol.110, no.12:31. (Kombucha Tea Mushroom for Diabetes?) 1988

Arauner, E. (In German): Der japanische Teepilz. Dtsch. Essigindustrie. vol.33, no.2:11-12. (The Japanese Tea Mushroom) 1929

Artz, Neal E., Osman, Elizabeth M. (In English): Biochemistry of Glucuronic Acid. New York Academic Press. New York. 1950

Bacinskaya, A.A. (In Russian): O rasprostranenii "cainogo kvassa" i Bacterium xylinum Brown. Zurnal Microbiologii. I:73-85. Petrograd. (On the distribution of "tea kvass" and Bacterium xylinum Brown.) 1914

Barbancik, G.F. (In Russian): Cainii grib i ego lecebnye svoistva. Izdame Tretye. Omsk: Omskoe oblastnoe kniznoe izdatelstvo. (The tea fungus and its therapeutic properties.) 1954

Bazarewski, S. (In German): Über den sogenannten "Wunderpilz" in den baltischen Provinzen. Correspondenzblatt Naturforscher-Verein. 57:61-69. Riga. (Concerning the "Miracle Mushroom" in the Baltic Provinces.) 1915

Bing, M. (In German): Heilwirkung des "Kombucha-schwammes". Umschau. 32:913-914. (Healing properties of the "Kombucha sponge.") 1928

Bing, M. (In German): Der Symbiont Bacterium xylinum—Schizosaccharomyces Pombe als Thera-peutikum. Die medizinische Welt. 2(42):1576-1577. (The Therapeutic Symbiosis of Bacterium Xyli-num—Schizosaccharomyces Pombe.) 1928

Bing, M. (In German): Zur Kombucha-frage. Die Umschau. 33(6):118-119. (On the Kombucha Question.) 1929

Brown, A.J. (In English): On an acetic Ferment which forms Cellulose. Journal of the Chemical Society. 49:432-439. London. 1886

Danielova, L.T. (In Russian): Bakteriostaticeskoe i baktericidnoe svoistvo nastoia "cainogo griba". Trudy Yerevanskogo zooverterinarnogo Instituta. 11:31-41. (The bacteriostatic and bactericidal properties of the "tea fungus" infusion.) 1949

Danielova, L.T. (In Russian): K morfologii "cainogo griba". Trudy Yerevanskogo zooverterinarnogo Instituta. 17:201-216. (Morphology of the "tea fungus.") 1954

Danielova, L.T. (In Russian): Biologiceskie osobennosti cainogo griba. Trudy Yerevanskogo zooverterinarnogo Instituta. 23:159-164. (The special biological characteristics of the tea fungus.) 1959

Dinslage, E., Ludorff, W. (In German): Der "indische Teepilz". Zeitschrift für Untersuchung der Lebensmittel. 53:458-467. (The "Indian Tea Mushroom.") 1927

Dutton, G.J. (In English): Glucuronic Acid. (GJD ed.) Academic Press. New York. 1966

Dutton, G.J. (In English): Glucuronidation of Drugs and Other Compounds. CRC Press, Boca Raton. 1980

Fasching, Rosina (Translated from German): Tea Fungus Kombucha, the Natural Remedy and its Significance in Cases of Cancer and other Metabolic Diseases.

Publisher: Wilhelm Ennsthaler, A-4402, Steyr, Austria. 1985

Filho, L.X., Paulo, M.Q., Pareira, E.C., Vicente, C. Phenolics from tea fungus analyzed by high performance liquid chromatography. Phyton (Buenos Aires). vol.45, no.2:187-191. 1985

Flück, V., Steinegger, E. (In German): Eine neue Hefekomponente des Teepilzes. Scientia pharmaceutica (Vienna). 25:43-44. (A New Yeast Component of Tea Mushrooms.) 1957

Foster, Daniel (In English): The Mushroom That Ate LA. Los Angeles Magazine. vol.39, no.11:118-124. Los Angeles. 1994

Frank, Günther (Translated from German): Kombucha, healthy beverage and natural remedy from the Far East, its correct preparation and use. Publisher: Wilhelm Ennsthaler, A-4402 Steyr, Austria. 1991

Funke, Hans (In German): Der Teepilz Kombucha. Natur & Heilen. 64:509-513. (The Tea Mushroom Kombucha.) 1987

Gadd, C.H. (In English): Tea Cider. Tea Quarterly (Talawakelle, Sri Lanka). 6:48-53. 1933

Gordienko, M. (In German): Review of a report (in Russian) by Utkin, L. Zbl. Bakt. 98,II:359. 1937

Haehn, H., Engel, M. (In German): Über die Bildung von Milchsäure durch Bacterium xylinum. Milchsäuregärung durch Kombucha. Zentralblatt für Bakteriologie, Mikrobiologie und Hygiene. II:182-185. (Concerning the formation of lactic acid through Bacterium xylinum. Latic acid formation through Kombucha.) 1929

Hahmann, C. (In German): Über Drogen und Drogenverfälschungen. Apotheker-Zeitung. vol.44, no. 37:561-563. 1929

Harms, H. (In German): Der japanische Teepilz. Therapeutische Berichte, Leverkusen. p.498-500. 1927

Henneberg, W. (In German): Zur Kenntnis der Schnellessig-und Weinessigbakterien. Zentralblatt für Bakteriologie. vol.17, no.25:789-804. 1907

Henneberg, W. (In German): Handbuch der Gärungsbakteriologie, Vol. 2 (Spezielle Pilzkunde, unter besonderer Berücksichtigung der Hefe-, Essig- und Milchsäurebakterien), 2nd edition. Verlag Paul Parey. Berlin 1926.

Hensler, P.O. (In German): Alles über Kombucha. Stutensee. (All About Kombucha.) 1989

Hermann, S. (In German): Über die sogenannte Kombucha. Biochemische Zeitschrift. 192:176-199. (About that which is called Kombucha.) 1928

Hermann, S. (In German): Die sogenannte "Kombucha." Umschau. 33:841-844. (That which is called Kombucha.) 1929

Hermann, S., Fodor, N. (In German): C-Vitamin-(1-Ascorbinsäure)-Bildung durch eine Symbiose von Essigbakterien und Hefen. Biochemische Z. vol.276, nos.5-6:323-325. (C-Vitamin {Ascorbic Acid} Formation through a Symbiosis of Vinegar Bacteria and Yeasts.) 1935

Hesseltine, Clifford W. (In English): A Millenium of Fungi, Food and Fermentation. Mycologia. 57:149-197. 1965

Irion, H. (In German): Fungus japonicus, Fungojapon Kombucha—Indisch-japanischer Teepilz. (IH ed.) Lehrgang für Drogistenfachschulen, Vol. 2 (Botanik/Drogenkunde), 4th edition. Verlagsgesellschaft Rudolf Müller. Eberswalde-Berlin-Leipsig. (Training Course for Pharmaceutical Technical Colleges.) 1944

Kaminski, Anette (In German): Ärzte: Pilz heilt Frauenleiden. Bild der Frau No. 2. Axel Springer Verlag. Hamburg. 1988

Kasevnik, L.L. (In Russian): Biohimia Vitamina C. Soobscenie III. O sposobnosti japonskogo cainogo griba sintezirovat' Vitamin C. — Bull. exp. Biol. i Med (Moscow) vol.3, no.1:87-88. [See **Schwaibold, N.**, for a review of this report.] (The biochemistry of vitamin C. 3rd report: The ability of the Japanese tea fungus to produce vitamin C.) 1937

Kobert, R. (In German): Der Kwass—ein unschädliches billiges Volkgetränk. 2nd edition. Haale a. d. Saale. 1913

Köhler, Valentin (In German): Glukuronsäure macht Krebspatienten Mut. Ärztliche Praxis. 33:887. (Glucuronic Acid Gives Cancer Patients Hope.) 1981

Köhler, Valentin, Köhler, J. (In German): Glukuronsäure als ökologische Hilfe. In the book: Sofortheilung des Waldes, Vol. 1, 2nd edition. (H. Kaegelmann ed.) Verlag zur heilen Welt. Windecke-Rosbach. (Glucuronic acid as an ecological aid.) 1985

Konovalov, I.N., Litvinov, M.A., Zakman, L.M. (In Russian): Izmenenie prirody i fiziologiceskii osobennostei cainogo griba (Medusomyces gisevii Lindau) v zavisimosti ot uslovii kultivirovania. Bit Zurnal (Moscow). vol.44, no.3:346-349. (Changes in the nature and physiological properties of the tea fungus (Medusomyces gisevii Lindau) regarding the requirements of the culture medium.) 1959

Körner, Helmut (In German): Der Teepilz Kombucha. Der Naturarzt. vol.108,no.5:14-16. (The Tea Mushroom Kombucha.) 1987

Körner, Helmut (In German): Kombucha-Zubereitung wurde von Sportmedizinern getestet. Natura-med (Neckarsulm). vol.4, no.10:592. (Kombucha preparation tested by sports physicians.) 1989

Kozaki, M., Koizumi, A., Kitagara, K. Microorganism of Zoogleal Mats Formed on Tea Decoction. J. Food Hyg. Soc. Japan. 13:89-96. 1972

Kraft, M.M. (In French): Le Champignon de Thé. Nova Hedwigia. vol.1, nos.3-4:297-304. (The Tea Mushroom.) 1959

Lakowitz, N. (In German): Teepilz und Teekwass. Apotheker-Zeitung. 43:298-300. 1928

Leskov, A.I. (In Russian): Novye svedenya o cainom gribe. Feldser i Akuerka (Moscow) vol.23, no.10:47-48. (New information about the tea fungus.) 1958

Lindau, G. (In German): Über Medusomyces Gisevii, eine neue Gattung und Art der Hefepilze. Ber. dt. bot. Ges. 31:243-248. (Concerning Medusomyces Gisevii, a New Genus and Spieces of Yeast Mushroom.) 1913

Lindner, P. (In German): Die vermeintliche neue Hefe Medusomyces Gisevii. Ber. dt. bot. Ges. 31:364-368. 1913

Lindner, P. (In German): Über Teekwass und Teekwasspilze. Mikrokosmos. 11:93-98. 1917

List, P.H., Hufschmidt, W. (In German): Basische Pilzinhaltsstoffe. 5. Mitteilung über biogene Amine und Aminosäuren des Teepilzes. Pharm. Zentralhalle. 98:593-598. 1959

Löwenheim, H. (In German): Über den indischen Teepilz. Apotheker-Zeitung. 42:148-149. (Concerning the Indian Tea Mushroom.) 1927

Mann, Ulrike (In German): Verblüffend—ein Pilz kuriert den Darm. Bild und Funk No. 35. Burda GmbH, Offenburg. (Amazing—a mushroom heals the intestines.) 1988

Matern, S., Bock, K.W., Gerok, W. (In English): Advances in Glucuronide Conjugation. (SM, KWB, WG ed.) MTP Press, Lancaster, United Kingdom. 1985

Meixner, A. (In German): Pilze selber züchten. Aarau (Switzerland). (Cultivating mushrooms yourself.) 1989

Merck Index (In English): Glucuronic Acid, p.701. Usnic Acid, p.1557. Eleventh Edition. 1989

Mollenda, L. (In German): Kombucha, ihre Heilbedeutung und Züchtung. Deutsche Essigindustrie. vol.32, no.27:243-244. (Kombucha, its healing properties and cultivation.) 1928

Mulder, D. (In English): A revival of tea cider. Tea Quarterly (Talawakelle, Sri Lanka). 32:48-53. 1961

Naumova, E.K. (In Russian): Meduzin—Novoe antibioticeskoe vescestvo, obrazumoe Medusomyces Gisevii. In: Vtoraya naucnaya Konferencia sanitarnogigieniceskogo fakulteta. 28-29 Aprelia 1949. Avtoreferati. p. 20-23. Kazan: Kazanskii gosudarstvenni medicinskii Institut. (Meduzin—a new antibiotic substance formed by Medusomyces Gisevii. In: second Scientific Conference of the Faculty of Health and Hygiene, April 28-29, 1949. Report p. 20-23. The Kazan State Medical Institute.) 1949

Paula Gomes, A. de (In Portuguese): Observações sobre a utilização de Zymomonas mobilis (Lindner) Kluyver et van Niel, 1936. (Thermobacterium mobile, Lindner 1928; Pseudomonas linderi Kluyver et Hoppen- brouwers, 1931), na Térapeutica Humana. Revista Instituto de Antibióticos (Pernambuco, Brazil). 2:77-81. 1959

People Magazine Staff (In English): Yeast Meets West. People Magazine. vol.43, no.6:192. 1995

Popiel, L.v. (In German): Zur Selbstherstellung von Essig. Pharmaz. Post (Vienna). vol.50, no.80:757-758. (On making vinegar oneself.) 1917

Reiss, Jürgen (In German): Der Teepilz und seine Stoffwechselprodukte. Deutsche Lebenmittel-Rundschau. vol.83, no.9:286-290. (The tea mushroom and its metabolic components.) 1987

Roots, H. (In Estonian): Teeseeneleotise Ravitoimest. Noukogude eesti tervishoid (Tallin, Estonia). 2:55-57. (The curative powers of the tea fungus.) 1959

Sakaryan, G.A., Danielova, L.T. (In Russian): Antibioticeskie svoistva nastoia griba Medusomyces gisevii (cainogo griba). Soobscenie 1. Trudy Yerevanskogo zooveterinarnogo Insttuta. 10:33-45. (The antibiotic capacities of the infusion of Meduso-myces gisevii (tea fungus). 1st Report.) 1948

Schröder, H. (In German): Teepilz und japanische Kristalle. Deine Gesundheit (Berlin). 7:29-30. 1989

Schwaibold, N. (In German): Review of a report (in Russian) by Kasevkik, L.D. Chem. Zbl. II:2860. 1937

Silva, R.L. de, Saravanapavan, T.V. (In English): Tea cider—a potential winner. Tea Quarterly (Talawakelle, Sri Lanka). 39:37-40. 1969

Sklenar, Rudolf (In German): Ein in der Iris sichtbarer Test für eine Stoffwechselstörung, kontrolliert an Hand von Dunkelfelduntersuchungen des Blutes nach Scheller. Erfahrungsheilkunde. vol.13,no.3. 1964

Sklenar, Rudolf (In German): Krebsdiagnose aus dem Blut und die Behandlung von Krebs, Präkanzerosen und sonstigen Stoffwechselkrankheiten mit der

Kombucha und Colipräparaten. Published by Fasching. Klagenfurt. (Cancer Diagnosis From Blood and the Treatment of Cancer and Pre-Cancerous Ailments by Means of Kombucha and Colicines.) 1983

Stadelmann, Eduard (In German): Der Teepilz—Eine Literaturzusammenstellung. Sydowia, Ann. mycolog. Ser. II. II:380-388. (The Tea Mushroom—A Compilation of Literature.) 1957

Stadelmann, Eduard (In German): Der Teepilz un seine antibiotische Wirkung. Zentralblatt Bakt. I. Abt. Ref. 180:401-435. (The Tea Mushroom and its Antibacterial Action.) 1961

Stark, J.B., Walter, E.D., Owens, H.S. (In English): Method of Isolation of Usnic Acid from *Ramalina reticulata*. Journal of the American Chemical Society. 72:1819-1820. 1950

Steiger, K.E., Steinegger, E. (In German): Über den Teepilz. Pharmaceutica Acta Helvetiae. 32:133-154. (Concerning the Tea Mushroom.) 1957

Sukiasyan, A.O. (In Russian): Vliyanie faktorov vnesnei sredy i istocnikov pitanya na nakoplenie antibioticeskii vescestv v kulture "cainogo griba". Soobscenie 1. Izucenie razlicnii fiziko-mehaniceskii vozodeistvii. Trudy Yerevanskogo zooveterinarnogo Instituta. 17:229-235. (The influence of culture milieu factors and nutrient sources on the accumulation of antibiotic substances in "tea fungus" cultures. 1st Report. The investigation of various physico-mechanical influen- ces.) 1954

Tea Export Bureau, Batavia (In English): Tea cider—a new drink in Java. Tea Quarterly (Talawakelle, Sri Lanka). 5:126-127. 1932

Tietze, Harald (In English): Kombucha, the Miracle Fungus. Publisher: H. Tietze, Bermagui Sth. NSW 2546 Australia. 1994

Utkin, L. (In Russian): O novom mikroorganizme iz gruppy uksusnyi bakterii. Mikrobiologia (Moscow). vol.6, no.4:421-434. [See Gordienko, M. for a review of this report.] (On a new micro-organism of the acetic acid group.) 1937

Valentin, H. (In German): Über die Verwendung des indischen Teepilzes und seine Gewinnung in trockener Form. Apotheker-Zeitung 43:1533-1536. 1928

Valentin, H. (In German): Wesentliche Bestandteile der Gärungsprodukte in den durch Pilztätigkeit gewonnenen Hausgetränken sowie die Verbreitung der letzteren. Apotheker-Zeitung. 45:1464-1465 and 1477-1478. (Essential components of fermentation products in the beverage gained by mushroom activity as well as its distribution.) 1930

Waldeck, H. (In German): Der Teepilz. Pharmazeutische Zentralhalle. 68:789-790. (The Tea Mushroom.) 1927

Wiechowski, W. (In German): Welche Stellung soll der Arzt zur Kombuchafrage einnehmen? Beiträge zur ärztlichen Fortbildung. 6:2-10. Prague. (What Position Should a Doctor Take on the Kombucha Question?) 1928

Yermolayeva, Z.V., Vaisberg, G.E., Afanaseyeva, T.I., Givenstal, N.I. (In Russian): O stimulyacii nekotorii antibakterialnii faktorov v organizme zitvotnii. Antibiotiki (Moscow). 3(6):46-50. (The stimulation of specific antibacterial factors in the animal organism.) 1958

Special thanks to Professor Stadelmann for many references, and to Lisa for helping to translate them.

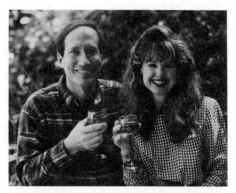

Sandy Holst & Betsy Pryor

THE LAST WORD

This book was carefully prepared using all the facts and information available to us about this remarkable health trend in the United States. We drew upon many previous studies and publications from other countries, which are gratefully acknowledged.

Since water, climate, cleanliness and other things affect the "growing" process, we can't guarantee the quality of the tea you make. But it's been grown for hundreds of years under a wide range of conditions, so you'll probably do fine.

Everyone's interested in their health and making the right decisions. We've tried to give the best possible information to help you, but obviously we can't make recommendations about anyone's particular medical case. Check with your health care provider.

Enjoy. Be happy. And healthy.

Betsy Pryor
Sanford Holst

INDEX

Get your own copy of
KOMBUCHA PHENOMENON

Or send one to a friend

It's as easy as . . .

1 Tell us where to send it:

Name _____

Address _____

City _____ State____Zip_____

If it's a gift, fill in your name:

It's a gift from

_____

2 And send a check or money order for

Book 11.95

Shipping .... __1.90__

$ 13.85

California residents add sales
tax for a total of **$ 14.85**

3 To: Sierra Sunrise Books,
14622 Ventura Blvd, Suite 800,
Sherman Oaks, CA 91403

(Allow 4-6 weeks for delivery)
(You may copy this order form)

B-1

Get your own copy of
KOMBUCHA PHENOMENON

Or send one to a friend

It's as easy as . . .

1 Tell us where to send it:

Name _____

Address _____

City _____ State ____ Zip _____

If it's a gift, fill in your name:

It's a gift from

_____

2 And send a check or money order for

Book 11.95
Shipping .... __1.90__
$ 13.85

California residents add sales
tax for a total of **$ 14.85**

3 To: Sierra Sunrise Books,
14622 Ventura Blvd, Suite 800,
Sherman Oaks, CA 91403

(Allow 4-6 weeks for delivery)
(You may copy this order form)   B-1